Nature's apothecary Quick Reference Guide to Topical Antibiotics

Luna Parnell

Table of Content

Introduction.. **3**
Legal Disclaimer... **5**
Topical Herbal Remedies.................................. 6
Universal Herbal Salve Recipe:.................... 7
Measurement Conversions......................... 10
Aloe Vera (Aloe barbadensis)......................... 12
Tea Tree (Melaleuca alternifolia)..................... 15
Calendula (Calendula officinalis)..................... 18
Lavender (Lavandula angustifolia)................... 21
Chamomile (Matricaria chamomilla).............. 25
Echinacea (Echinacea purpurea).................... 28
Rosemary (Rosmarinus officinalis)................. 32
Myrrh (Commiphora myrrha)......................... 36
Garlic (Allium sativum)...................................39
Goldenseal (Hydrastis canadensis)..................44
Marigold (Calendula officinalis)..................... 48
Comfrey (Symphytum officinale)....................52
Hyssop (Hyssopus officinalis)........................55
Lemon Balm (Melissa officinalis)................... 58
Mullein (Verbascum thapsus)......................... 61
Plantain (Plantago major)...............................64
St. John's Wort (Hypericum perforatum)........67
Yarrow (Achillea millefolium)........................70

Introduction

Welcome to *Nature's Apothecary: A Quick Reference Guide to Topical Antibiotics*, your essential companion for harnessing the power of herbal remedies in managing skin infections, burns, cuts, and acne naturally. In this comprehensive guide, we explore the therapeutic potential of various herbs renowned for their antibacterial properties. Each herb discussed here offers a natural alternative rooted in traditional medicine, providing holistic solutions for maintaining healthy, radiant skin.

Discover the soothing benefits of Aloe Vera, the potent antimicrobial properties of Tea Tree, and the calming effects of Lavender and Calendula. Learn how these herbs can alleviate skin irritations, accelerate wound healing, and combat bacterial infections effectively. Whether you're seeking relief from minor burns, cuts, acne flare-ups, or other skin conditions, this guide equips you with practical insights and easy-to-follow recipes for creating herbal preparations like infused oils, salves, and compresses.

Empower yourself with the knowledge to cultivate a natural skincare regimen using Nature's Apothecary. Enhance your understanding of each herb's scientific benefits, optimal dosage recommendations, and methods for safe and effective application. Embrace the wisdom of centuries-old herbal remedies and integrate them seamlessly into your daily routine for healthier, resilient skin.

Join us on a journey through *Nature's Apothecary*, where ancient wisdom meets modern skincare, offering you a reliable toolkit for nurturing your skin and promoting well-being through the therapeutic wonders of herbal topical antibiotics.

Legal Disclaimer

The information provided in this book is for educational purposes only and is not intended as medical advice. Readers are advised to consult with a qualified healthcare professional regarding the use of medicinal plants and herbs, especially if pregnant, nursing, taking medication, or have a medical condition. The author and publisher do not advocate self-diagnosis or self-medication and disclaim any liability arising from the misuse of information contained herein.

While every effort has been made to ensure the accuracy of the information presented, herbal remedies and their effects may vary based on individual circumstances. It is recommended to conduct thorough research and exercise caution when preparing and using herbal remedies. The FDA (Food and Drug Administration) has not evaluated the statements made in this book. These products are not intended to diagnose, treat, cure, or prevent any disease.

Topical Herbal Remedies

Exploring the healing potential of medicinal plants through topical applications offers a direct and effective approach to managing various skin conditions and localized infections. This section of the book delves into the art and science of preparing herbal remedies for external use, focusing on ointments, creams, poultices, and other topical forms that harness the antibiotic properties of nature's apothecary.

Medicinal plants have a long history of being revered for their ability to heal and protect the skin. From the soothing properties of aloe vera (Aloe barbadensis) to the potent antimicrobial effects of tea tree (Melaleuca alternifolia), each plant profiled here offers a unique blend of active compounds—whether anti-inflammatory, antibacterial, or wound-healing—that contribute to their therapeutic benefits.

This section equips you with practical knowledge on creating herbal ointments to soothe burns, formulating healing creams for conditions like eczema and psoriasis, and preparing poultices for treating wounds and infections. Step-by-step instructions, recipes, and tips on selecting, preparing, and applying herbal remedies effectively are provided to ensure you can integrate herbal medicine into your daily life confidently.

Whether you're seeking relief from minor skin irritations or aiming to enhance your skincare routine with natural ingredients, this section empowers you with the tools to explore the rich tradition and modern applications of topical herbal remedies. Discover how these natural solutions can support optimal skin health and well-being, ensuring safe and effective use for a holistic approach to healing.

Universal Herbal Salve Recipe:

Ingredients:

- 1 cup carrier oil (such as olive oil, coconut oil, or almond oil)
- 1/4 cup beeswax pellets or grated beeswax
- 1/4 cup dried herbs of your choice (e.g., calendula flowers, lavender, chamomile, comfrey, plantain, etc.)

- Optional: a few drops of essential oil for fragrance (e.g., lavender, tea tree, or peppermint)

Equipment:

- Double boiler or heat-safe bowl and saucepan
- Fine mesh strainer or cheesecloth
- Heat-resistant container or jars for storing the salve

Instructions:

1. **Infusing the Oil:**
   - In a double boiler or a heat-safe bowl placed over a saucepan with water, combine the carrier oil and dried herbs.
   - Heat gently over low to medium heat for 1-2 hours, stirring occasionally. Ensure the oil does not boil.
   - Alternatively, use a slow cooker on low heat for 4-6 hours or leave the mixture in a sunny spot for a few weeks for a solar-infused oil.
2. **Straining the Oil:**
   - Once infused, strain the oil using a fine mesh strainer or

cheesecloth into a clean bowl or container. Squeeze out as much oil as possible from the herbs.

3. **Making the Salve:**
   - Return the infused oil to the double boiler or heat-safe bowl.
   - Add the beeswax pellets or grated beeswax to the infused oil.
   - Heat gently over low heat until the beeswax is completely melted, stirring occasionally to combine well.
   - Optional: Add a few drops of essential oil for fragrance, if desired, and stir to incorporate.

4. **Pouring and Cooling:**
   - Carefully pour the melted salve mixture into heat-resistant containers or jars.
   - Allow the salve to cool and solidify at room temperature. This may take a few hours, depending on the size of your containers.

5. **Storage and Use:**
   - Once cooled and solidified, label and store your herbal salve in a cool, dry place away from direct sunlight.

- To use, apply a small amount of salve to clean, dry skin as needed for soothing and healing properties.

The herbs used can vary based on your intended use (e.g., antibacterial, anti-inflammatory, soothing). Adjust the strength by increasing or decreasing the amount of herbs used in the infusion process. Always perform a small patch test before widespread use, especially if you have sensitive skin or allergies.

This universal herbal salve recipe allows for customization with a variety of herbs known for their healing properties, making it versatile for different skin conditions and needs.

Measurement Conversions

Volume Measurements:

- 1 teaspoon (tsp) = 5 milliliters (ml)
- 1 tablespoon (Tbsp) = 3 teaspoons = 15 ml
- 1 fluid ounce (fl oz) = 2 tablespoons = 30 ml
- 1 cup = 8 fluid ounces = 240 ml

- 1 pint (pt) = 2 cups = 16 fluid ounces = 480 ml
- 1 quart (qt) = 2 pints = 4 cups = 32 fluid ounces = 960 ml
- 1 gallon (gal) = 4 quarts = 16 cups = 128 fluid ounces = 3.785 liters

Weight Measurements:

- 1 ounce (oz) = 28.35 grams (g)
- 1 pound (lb) = 16 ounces = 453.59 grams

Metric to Imperial Conversions:

- 1 milliliter (ml) = 0.034 fluid ounces
- 1 liter (l) = 1.0567 quarts = 33.814 fluid ounces
- 1 gram (g) = 0.0353 ounces
- 1 kilogram (kg) = 2.2046 pounds

Common Herbal Measurement:

- 1 part (by volume) = Any unit of measurement (e.g., teaspoon, cup) that can be used to measure herbs

Aloe Vera (Aloe barbadensis)

Description: Aloe vera, a member of the succulent family, is widely recognized for its spiky, fleshy leaves that contain a clear gel-like substance. Native to North Africa, Southern Europe, and the Canary Islands, this plant has a long history of medicinal use dating back to ancient civilizations like the Egyptians, Greeks, and Romans. Its popularity continues today due to its therapeutic benefits for skin health.

Scientific Benefits: The gel inside aloe vera leaves is rich in bioactive compounds, including polysaccharides, glycoproteins, vitamins (such as vitamin A, C, and E), minerals (including calcium, magnesium, and zinc), and enzymes (such as bradykinase). These components contribute to its multifaceted healing properties:

- **Anti-inflammatory:** Aloe vera helps reduce inflammation, making it beneficial for conditions like sunburns, acne, and dermatitis.
- **Wound Healing:** It promotes wound healing by stimulating collagen synthesis and enhancing the formation of new blood vessels (angiogenesis).

- **Antioxidant:** The antioxidants in aloe vera help neutralize free radicals, protecting skin cells from oxidative stress and premature aging.

Antibacterial Properties: Aloe vera exhibits potent antibacterial activity against various pathogens, including bacteria such as Staphylococcus aureus, Streptococcus pyogenes, and Pseudomonas aeruginosa. The antibacterial effects are primarily attributed to compounds like anthraquinones (e.g., aloin and emodin) and saponins (e.g., glycosides such as barbaloin).

Types of Infections Targeted: Aloe vera is effective in treating a range of skin infections and conditions:

- **Burns:** It provides cooling relief and accelerates healing in minor burns, including sunburns.
- **Cuts and Wounds:** Aloe vera's antimicrobial properties help prevent infections and promote faster healing of cuts, abrasions, and surgical wounds.
- **Acne:** Its anti-inflammatory and antibacterial actions can reduce acne symptoms and aid in healing acne lesions.

- **Psoriasis and Eczema:** Aloe vera's soothing properties help alleviate itching and irritation associated with psoriasis and eczema.

Dosage Recommendations: For topical use, apply a thin layer of aloe vera gel directly to the affected area 2-3 times daily. It can be used alone as a gel or incorporated into formulations like creams and ointments for enhanced moisturization and healing effects.

Preparation Recipe: *Simple Aloe Vera Gel Application:*

1. **Harvesting and Processing:** Select a mature leaf from the aloe vera plant. To eliminate the yellow latex (which can be irritating), allow the leaf to stand upright for 10-15 minutes after cutting.
2. **Extracting the Gel:** Slice the leaf open lengthwise and scoop out the clear gel using a spoon. Collect the gel in a clean container.
3. **Application:** Apply the fresh gel directly onto clean, dry skin. Gently massage until absorbed. For optimal results, repeat application 2-3 times daily.

Tea Tree (Melaleuca alternifolia)

Description: Tea tree, also known as Melaleuca alternifolia, is an evergreen tree native to Australia. It is renowned for its small, narrow leaves and papery bark. The essential oil extracted from tea tree leaves has been used for centuries in traditional Aboriginal medicine for its powerful medicinal properties.

Scientific Benefits: Tea tree essential oil contains several bioactive compounds, primarily terpinen-4-ol, which is responsible for its antimicrobial and anti-inflammatory effects. It also contains other terpenes like cineole, pinene, and terpinolene, contributing to its therapeutic benefits.

Antibacterial Properties: Tea tree oil is well-known for its potent antibacterial properties. It exhibits activity against a wide range of bacteria, including Staphylococcus aureus, Streptococcus pyogenes, and Escherichia coli. The primary mechanism of action involves disrupting bacterial cell membranes and inhibiting bacterial growth.

Types of Infections Targeted: Tea tree oil is effective in treating various skin infections and conditions:

- **Acne:** Its anti-inflammatory and antibacterial properties help reduce acne-causing bacteria (Propionibacterium acnes) and inflammation associated with acne.
- **Athlete's Foot:** Tea tree oil's antifungal properties can help alleviate symptoms of athlete's foot, including itching, scaling, and discomfort.
- **Minor Cuts and Wounds:** It can be applied topically to minor cuts and wounds to prevent infection and promote healing.
- **Fungal Infections:** Tea tree oil is effective against fungal infections like nail fungus (onychomycosis) and ringworm.

Dosage Recommendations: Tea tree oil should be diluted before topical application to prevent skin irritation, especially for sensitive skin. A typical dilution is 1-2 drops of tea tree oil per teaspoon of carrier oil (such as coconut oil or almond oil). Apply a small amount to the affected area 1-2 times daily.

Preparation Recipe: *Tea Tree Oil Antiseptic Ointment:*

1. **Ingredients:**
   - 1/4 cup coconut oil (solid form)
   - 10-15 drops tea tree essential oil
2. **Preparation:**
   - In a small bowl, mix the coconut oil and tea tree essential oil until well combined.
   - Store the mixture in a clean, airtight container.
3. **Application:**
   - Cleanse the affected area thoroughly.
   - Apply a small amount of the tea tree oil ointment directly to the skin using clean fingertips.
   - Massage gently until absorbed. Reapply 1-2 times daily or as needed.

Calendula (Calendula officinalis)

Description: Calendula, also known as pot marigold, is a bright and cheerful flowering plant belonging to the Asteraceae family. Native to the Mediterranean region, calendula is prized not only for its ornamental beauty but also for its medicinal properties. It produces vibrant yellow or orange flowers with a slightly spicy aroma.

Scientific Benefits: Calendula contains numerous active compounds, including flavonoids (e.g., quercetin and rutin), triterpene saponins (e.g., calendulosides), and carotenoids (e.g., lutein and beta-carotene). These constituents contribute to its anti-inflammatory, antimicrobial, and wound-healing properties. Calendula also exhibits antioxidant effects, protecting cells from oxidative stress.

Antibacterial Properties: Calendula possesses broad-spectrum antibacterial activity, making it effective against various bacteria, including Staphylococcus aureus and Streptococcus pyogenes. Its antimicrobial action helps prevent infection and promotes healing in wounds and skin irritations.

Types of Infections Targeted: Calendula is beneficial for treating a range of skin infections and conditions:

- **Wounds and Cuts:** It accelerates wound healing by promoting tissue regeneration and reducing inflammation.
- **Minor Burns:** Calendula soothes and moisturizes burned skin while preventing bacterial growth.
- **Eczema and Dermatitis:** Its anti-inflammatory properties help relieve itching and inflammation associated with eczema and dermatitis.
- **Acne:** Calendula's antimicrobial effects can help reduce acne-causing bacteria and calm acne-prone skin.

Dosage Recommendations: Calendula can be used topically in various forms, including creams, ointments, and infused oils. For general use, apply a calendula-infused oil or cream to the affected area 2-3 times daily. It is generally well-tolerated, but individuals with sensitive skin should perform a patch test first.

Preparation Recipe: *Calendula Infused Oil:*

1. **Ingredients:**

- Dried calendula flowers
- Carrier oil (such as olive oil, almond oil, or coconut oil)

2. **Preparation:**
   - Fill a clean glass jar halfway with dried calendula flowers.
   - Cover the flowers completely with your chosen carrier oil.
   - Seal the jar tightly and place it in a warm, sunny spot for 4-6 weeks to infuse. Alternatively, use a double boiler to gently heat the mixture for 1-2 hours, then strain.

3. **Application:**
   - Strain the infused oil through a fine mesh strainer or cheesecloth into a clean container.
   - Store the calendula-infused oil in a cool, dark place. Use it as a base for creams, lotions, or apply directly to the skin as needed for its healing and soothing benefits.

This calendula-infused oil recipe allows you to harness the herb's antibacterial and healing properties effectively, making it a versatile addition to your skincare routine.

Lavender (Lavandula angustifolia)

Description: Lavender, known scientifically as Lavandula angustifolia, is a fragrant perennial herb belonging to the Lamiaceae family. Native to the Mediterranean region, lavender is prized for its beautiful purple flowers and distinctive aroma. It has been used for centuries in traditional medicine, aromatherapy, and culinary applications.

Scientific Benefits: Lavender contains several bioactive compounds, including linalool, linalyl acetate, and camphor. These constituents impart lavender with anti-inflammatory, antimicrobial, and antioxidant properties. Lavender essential oil is particularly renowned for its calming effects on the nervous system and its ability to promote relaxation.

Antibacterial Properties: Lavender essential oil exhibits significant antibacterial activity against various pathogens, including both Gram-positive (e.g., Staphylococcus aureus) and Gram-negative (e.g., Escherichia coli) bacteria. Its antibacterial effects are attributed to the presence of compounds like linalool and linalyl acetate, which disrupt bacterial cell membranes and inhibit bacterial growth.

Types of Infections Targeted: Lavender is effective in treating and preventing various skin infections and conditions:

- **Acne:** Its antimicrobial and anti-inflammatory properties help reduce acne-causing bacteria (Propionibacterium acnes) and soothe inflamed skin.
- **Minor Cuts and Wounds:** Lavender accelerates wound healing by promoting cellular regeneration and reducing inflammation.
- **Dermatitis and Eczema:** Its calming effects can alleviate itching and inflammation associated with dermatitis and eczema.
- **Fungal Infections:** Lavender oil's antifungal properties can help combat fungal infections like athlete's foot and nail fungus.

Dosage Recommendations: Lavender essential oil should be diluted before topical application to avoid skin irritation, especially for sensitive skin types. A safe dilution ratio is typically 1-2 drops of lavender oil per teaspoon of carrier oil (such as coconut oil or almond oil). Apply the diluted mixture to the affected area 2-3 times daily.

Preparation Recipe: *Lavender Infused Salve:*

1. **Ingredients:**
    - 1/2 cup dried lavender flowers
    - 1 cup carrier oil (e.g., olive oil, sweet almond oil)
    - 1/4 cup beeswax pellets
    - Optional: 10-15 drops lavender essential oil (for added fragrance and potency)
2. **Preparation:**
    - In a clean, dry glass jar, combine the dried lavender flowers and carrier oil.
    - Seal the jar tightly and place it in a warm, sunny spot for 4-6 weeks to infuse. Shake the jar gently every few days to ensure the flowers are fully submerged.
3. **Straining and Melting:**
    - After infusion, strain the lavender-infused oil through a fine mesh strainer or cheesecloth into a clean bowl.

- In a double boiler, melt the beeswax pellets over low heat. Once melted, add the lavender-infused oil and stir well to combine. Remove from heat.

4. **Cooling and Storing:**
    - Pour the mixture into clean, sterilized containers (such as jars or tins) and let it cool completely at room temperature until solidified.

5. **Application:**
    - Use the lavender-infused salve as needed for its antibacterial and soothing properties. Apply a small amount to clean, dry skin and massage gently until absorbed.

Chamomile (Matricaria chamomilla)

Description: Chamomile, scientifically known as Matricaria chamomilla or Matricaria recutita, is a daisy-like flowering herb belonging to the Asteraceae family. It is native to Europe and Western Asia but is now cultivated worldwide for its medicinal and aromatic properties. Chamomile flowers resemble small daisies with white petals and a yellow center. The plant has a gentle, apple-like scent and is commonly used in herbal teas, skincare products, and topical preparations.

Scientific Benefits: Chamomile contains various bioactive compounds, including chamazulene, alpha-bisabolol, flavonoids (e.g., apigenin and luteolin), and essential oils (such as bisabolol oxide). These constituents contribute to chamomile's anti-inflammatory, antioxidant, and antimicrobial properties.

Antibacterial Properties: Chamomile exhibits mild antibacterial activity against both Gram-positive (e.g., Staphylococcus aureus) and Gram-negative (e.g., Escherichia coli) bacteria. Its antibacterial effects are attributed to compounds like chamazulene and alpha-bisabolol, which help inhibit bacterial growth and reduce inflammation.

Types of Infections Targeted: Chamomile is effective in treating various skin infections and conditions:

- **Skin Irritations:** It soothes and calms irritated skin, making it beneficial for conditions like eczema, dermatitis, and sunburns.
- **Minor Wounds and Cuts:** Chamomile promotes wound healing by reducing inflammation and preventing infection.
- **Acne:** Its anti-inflammatory and antibacterial properties can help reduce acne symptoms and prevent breakouts.
- **Allergic Skin Reactions:** Chamomile's soothing properties can alleviate itching and redness caused by allergic reactions.

Dosage Recommendations: Chamomile can be used topically in various forms, including infused oils, creams, and compresses. For topical application, prepare chamomile-infused oil by steeping dried chamomile flowers in a carrier oil (such as olive oil or almond oil) for 4-6 weeks. Apply the infused oil to the affected area 2-3 times daily or as needed.

Preparation Recipe: *Chamomile Infused Oil:*

1. **Ingredients:**
   - 1/2 cup dried chamomile flowers
   - 1 cup carrier oil (e.g., olive oil, sweet almond oil)
2. **Preparation:**
   - Place the dried chamomile flowers in a clean, dry glass jar.
   - Cover the flowers completely with your chosen carrier oil.
   - Seal the jar tightly and place it in a warm, sunny spot for 4-6 weeks to infuse. Shake the jar gently every few days to ensure the flowers are fully submerged.
3. **Straining and Storing:**
   - After infusion, strain the chamomile-infused oil through a fine mesh strainer or cheesecloth into a clean container.
   - Store the infused oil in a cool, dark place. Use it as a base for creams, lotions, or apply directly to the skin as needed for its soothing and antibacterial benefits.

Echinacea (Echinacea purpurea)

Description: Echinacea, scientifically known as Echinacea purpurea, is a flowering plant in the Asteraceae family. Native to North America, it is commonly referred to as purple coneflower due to its distinctive daisy-like purple petals and prominent cone-shaped center. Echinacea has been traditionally used by Native American tribes for its medicinal properties, and today it is widely recognized for its immune-boosting benefits.

Scientific Benefits: Echinacea contains active compounds such as alkamides, polysaccharides, flavonoids (e.g., quercetin and rutin), and caffeic acid derivatives. These constituents contribute to echinacea's immunostimulant, anti-inflammatory, and antioxidant properties. Echinacea is known for its ability to enhance immune function and support overall health.

Antibacterial Properties: Echinacea exhibits moderate antibacterial activity against a range of bacteria, including both Gram-positive (e.g., Staphylococcus aureus) and Gram-negative (e.g., Escherichia coli) bacteria. Its antibacterial effects are attributed to compounds like echinacoside and alkamides, which help inhibit bacterial growth and enhance immune response.

Types of Infections Targeted: Echinacea is beneficial for treating various infections and promoting wound healing:

- **Respiratory Infections:** It can help reduce the severity and duration of common colds, flu, and upper respiratory infections.
- **Skin Infections:** Echinacea's antibacterial properties support the treatment of minor skin infections, cuts, and wounds.
- **Urinary Tract Infections (UTIs):** It may aid in alleviating symptoms and promoting recovery from UTIs by combating bacterial growth.

Dosage Recommendations: Echinacea is available in various forms, including capsules, extracts, and topical preparations. For topical use, echinacea extract or oil can be applied directly to the skin. Follow product-specific instructions or consult with a healthcare provider for appropriate dosage recommendations.

Preparation Recipe: *Echinacea Infused Oil:*

1. **Ingredients:**
   - 1/2 cup dried echinacea root or flowers
   - 1 cup carrier oil (e.g., olive oil, jojoba oil)
2. **Preparation:**
   - Place the dried echinacea root or flowers in a clean, dry glass jar.
   - Cover the herbs completely with your chosen carrier oil.
   - Seal the jar tightly and place it in a warm, sunny spot for 4-6 weeks to infuse. Shake the jar gently every few days to ensure the herbs are fully submerged.
3. **Straining and Storing:**
   - After infusion, strain the echinacea-infused oil through a fine mesh strainer or cheesecloth into a clean container.
   - Store the infused oil in a cool, dark place. Use it as a base for creams, lotions, or apply directly to the skin as needed for its antibacterial and healing benefits.

This echinacea-infused oil recipe allows you to harness the herb's antibacterial properties effectively, making it a versatile addition to your natural skincare routine and first aid kit.

Rosemary (Rosmarinus officinalis)

Description: Rosemary, scientifically known as Rosmarinus officinalis, is an aromatic evergreen shrub belonging to the Lamiaceae family. Native to the Mediterranean region, rosemary is characterized by its needle-like leaves and small, blue-purple flowers. It has a woody aroma with hints of pine and citrus, making it a popular culinary herb and valued for its medicinal properties.

Scientific Benefits: Rosemary contains several bioactive compounds, including rosmarinic acid, caffeic acid derivatives, flavonoids (e.g., luteolin), and essential oils (e.g., cineole). These constituents contribute to rosemary's antioxidant, anti-inflammatory, and antimicrobial properties. Rosemary is known for its stimulating and invigorating effects on both the body and mind.

Antibacterial Properties: Rosemary essential oil exhibits strong antibacterial activity against various pathogens, including both Gram-positive (e.g., Staphylococcus aureus) and Gram-negative (e.g., Escherichia coli) bacteria. Its antibacterial effects are primarily attributed to compounds like cineole

and rosmarinic acid, which help inhibit
bacterial growth and promote skin health.

Types of Infections Targeted: Rosemary is
effective in treating and preventing various
skin infections and conditions:

- **Acne:** Its antimicrobial properties can
  help reduce acne-causing bacteria
  (Propionibacterium acnes) and balance
  oily skin.
- **Dermatitis and Eczema:** Rosemary's
  anti-inflammatory effects can soothe
  itching and irritation associated with
  dermatitis and eczema.
- **Minor Cuts and Wounds:** It
  promotes wound healing by accelerating
  skin regeneration and preventing
  infection.
- **Scalp Conditions:** Rosemary oil is
  used to improve scalp health, combat
  dandruff, and promote hair growth.

Dosage Recommendations: Rosemary
essential oil should be diluted before topical
application to prevent skin irritation, especially
for sensitive skin. A safe dilution ratio is
typically 1-2 drops of rosemary oil per teaspoon
of carrier oil (such as coconut oil or jojoba oil).

Apply the diluted mixture to the affected area 2-3 times daily or as needed.

Preparation Recipe: *Rosemary Infused Vinegar:*

1. **Ingredients:**
    - 1 cup fresh rosemary sprigs (or 1/2 cup dried rosemary)
    - 2 cups apple cider vinegar (or white vinegar)
2. **Preparation:**
    - Place the rosemary sprigs (or dried rosemary) in a clean glass jar.
    - Heat the vinegar in a saucepan until it reaches a simmer. Pour the hot vinegar over the rosemary in the jar, covering the herbs completely.
3. **Steeping and Straining:**
    - Seal the jar tightly and let it steep for 2-4 weeks in a cool, dark place, shaking the jar gently every few days.
    - After steeping, strain the infused vinegar through a fine mesh strainer or cheesecloth into a clean container.
4. **Application:**

- Dilute the rosemary-infused vinegar with water (1 part vinegar to 2 parts water) for use as a skin toner or hair rinse.
- Apply the diluted vinegar to the skin with a cotton ball to cleanse and tone, or use as a final hair rinse after shampooing to promote scalp health and shine.

This rosemary-infused vinegar recipe harnesses the herb's antibacterial and astringent properties, making it a beneficial addition to your skincare and hair care regimen.

Myrrh (Commiphora myrrha)

Description: Myrrh, derived from the resin of the Commiphora myrrha tree, is a small thorny tree or shrub native to regions of Arabia, Ethiopia, and Somalia. It has been valued for centuries for its medicinal properties and use in perfumery. Myrrh resin is dark reddish-brown with a rich, aromatic fragrance.

Scientific Benefits: Myrrh contains bioactive compounds such as furanosesquiterpenes, terpenoids, and phenolic acids, which contribute to its antioxidant, anti-inflammatory, and antimicrobial properties. These constituents make myrrh effective in promoting wound healing and combating infections.

Antibacterial Properties: Myrrh resin exhibits potent antibacterial activity against a broad spectrum of bacteria, including both Gram-positive (e.g., Staphylococcus aureus) and Gram-negative (e.g., Escherichia coli) strains. Its antibacterial effects help prevent infections and support skin health.

Types of Infections Targeted: Myrrh is beneficial for treating various topical infections and promoting wound healing:

- **Wound Care:** Applied topically, myrrh helps cleanse wounds, reduce inflammation, and promote tissue regeneration.
- **Skin Irritations:** It soothes and protects irritated skin, making it useful for conditions like eczema, dermatitis, and minor burns.
- **Oral Health:** Myrrh-infused oils or ointments are used for oral hygiene to combat gum disease and oral infections.

Dosage Recommendations: For topical applications, myrrh resin can be used in various forms, including infused oils, salves, or ointments. Dilute myrrh essential oil or tincture in a carrier oil (such as coconut oil or olive oil) before applying to the skin. Follow product-specific instructions or consult with a healthcare provider for appropriate dosage recommendations.

Preparation Recipe: *Myrrh Infused Oil:*

1. **Ingredients:**
   - 1/4 cup myrrh resin powder (or small resin pieces)
   - 1 cup carrier oil (e.g., olive oil, almond oil)
2. **Preparation:**

- In a clean, dry glass jar, combine the myrrh resin with the carrier oil.
- Seal the jar tightly and place it in a warm, sunny spot for 4-6 weeks to infuse. Shake the jar gently every few days to ensure the resin is fully submerged.

3. **Straining and Storing:**
   - After infusion, strain the myrrh-infused oil through a fine mesh strainer or cheesecloth into a clean container.
   - Store the infused oil in a cool, dark place. Use it as a base for ointments or apply directly to the skin as needed for its antibacterial and healing properties.

Garlic (Allium sativum)

Description: Garlic, scientifically known as Allium sativum, is a bulbous plant renowned for both its culinary and medicinal uses. Originating from Central Asia, garlic has a long history of cultivation and consumption dating back thousands of years. It belongs to the Allium genus, which includes other familiar members like onions, leeks, and shallots. Characterized by its pungent aroma and distinctive flavor, garlic is prized not only for its culinary versatility but also for its potent medicinal properties.

Scientific Benefits: Garlic is rich in bioactive compounds, notably allicin, diallyl disulfide, S-allyl cysteine, and various sulfur compounds. These compounds contribute to garlic's diverse health benefits, including its potent antimicrobial, anti-inflammatory, and antioxidant properties. Allicin, formed when garlic is crushed or chopped, is particularly noted for its antibacterial effects. It works by disrupting bacterial cell membranes and inhibiting their growth, making garlic a valuable natural remedy for combating infections.

Antibacterial Properties: Garlic demonstrates robust antibacterial activity against a wide range of bacteria, encompassing both Gram-positive (e.g., Staphylococcus aureus) and Gram-negative (e.g., Escherichia coli) strains. This broad spectrum of action is attributed to allicin and other sulfur-containing compounds present in garlic, which effectively target bacterial pathogens. By interfering with bacterial cell processes and membrane integrity, garlic helps prevent infections and supports the body's natural defenses.

Types of Infections Targeted: Garlic is beneficial for treating various topical infections and promoting skin health:

- **Skin Infections:** Topically applied garlic can aid in treating fungal infections such as athlete's foot and nail fungus due to its potent antifungal properties. It helps inhibit the growth of fungi responsible for these conditions, promoting faster healing.
- **Acne:** Its antibacterial and anti-inflammatory properties make garlic beneficial for managing acne. It can help reduce the population of acne-causing bacteria (Propionibacterium acnes) on the skin

and alleviate inflammation, contributing to clearer and healthier skin.

- **Wound Healing:** Garlic supports wound healing processes by reducing inflammation, protecting against infection, and promoting tissue repair. Applied topically to minor cuts, scrapes, and abrasions, garlic helps cleanse wounds and accelerate healing.

Dosage Recommendations: For topical applications, garlic can be utilized in various forms:

- **Garlic Infused Oil:** Prepare by infusing crushed or finely chopped garlic cloves in a carrier oil such as olive oil or coconut oil. Allow the mixture to sit for several weeks to extract the beneficial compounds from garlic. The infused oil can then be applied directly to the skin as needed to promote healing and combat infections.
- **Garlic Paste:** Create a paste by crushing fresh garlic cloves and applying it directly to affected areas of the skin. Leave the paste on for a brief period before rinsing off to avoid potential irritation, ensuring it remains effective in treating localized infections.

Preparation Recipe: *Garlic Infused Oil:*

1. **Ingredients:**
   - 3-4 garlic cloves, peeled and finely chopped
   - 1/2 cup carrier oil (e.g., olive oil, coconut oil)
2. **Preparation:**
   - Heat the carrier oil gently in a small saucepan over low heat.
   - Add the finely chopped garlic cloves to the warmed oil, allowing them to infuse together for approximately 5-10 minutes. Stir occasionally to ensure even distribution and prevent burning.
   - Remove the saucepan from heat and let the garlic-infused oil cool to room temperature.
3. **Straining and Storing:**
   - Once cooled, strain the infused oil through a fine mesh strainer or cheesecloth into a clean, airtight container.
   - Store the garlic-infused oil in a cool, dark place to maintain its potency and effectiveness. Use it topically as part of your skincare regimen or for treating minor skin infections, applying a small

amount directly to the affected
area.

This garlic-infused oil recipe provides a natural and versatile solution for harnessing garlic's potent antibacterial and healing properties in topical applications. By incorporating garlic into your skincare routine, you can promote skin health, support wound healing, and combat various skin infections effectively.

Goldenseal (Hydrastis canadensis)

Description: Goldenseal, scientifically known as Hydrastis canadensis, is a perennial herb native to the eastern United States and Canada. It belongs to the Ranunculaceae family and is characterized by its small, wrinkled rhizomes and thick, yellow roots. Goldenseal has a long history of traditional use by Native American tribes for its medicinal properties, particularly as a natural antibiotic and immune system enhancer.

Scientific Benefits: Goldenseal contains bioactive alkaloids, primarily berberine, hydrastine, and canadine, which contribute to its medicinal properties. Berberine, in particular, is known for its potent antimicrobial, anti-inflammatory, and immune-stimulating effects. These compounds make goldenseal valuable for supporting immune function and combating various infections.

Antibacterial Properties: Goldenseal exhibits strong antibacterial activity against both Gram-positive (e.g., Staphylococcus aureus) and Gram-negative (e.g., Escherichia coli) bacteria. The alkaloids berberine and hydrastine are responsible for these antibacterial effects, disrupting bacterial cell membranes and inhibiting their growth.

Types of Infections Targeted: Goldenseal is effective in treating and preventing various topical infections and supporting overall skin health:

- **Skin Infections:** Applied topically, goldenseal ointments or creams can help treat minor cuts, wounds, and skin infections. Its antimicrobial properties aid in reducing bacterial growth and promoting healing.
- **Eye Infections:** Goldenseal is sometimes used in eye wash solutions to alleviate symptoms of conjunctivitis (pink eye) and other eye infections.
- **Mouth and Throat Infections:** It is used in mouthwashes or gargles to support oral hygiene and treat infections like gingivitis and sore throat.

Dosage Recommendations: For topical applications, goldenseal can be used in various forms:

- **Goldenseal Ointment:** Apply a thin layer of goldenseal ointment directly to affected areas of the skin, such as cuts or wounds, 2-3 times daily.

- **Goldenseal Infused Oil:** Create an infused oil by steeping dried goldenseal root in a carrier oil (e.g., olive oil or jojoba oil) for several weeks. Apply the infused oil topically to promote healing and combat infections.

Preparation Recipe: *Goldenseal Infused Oil:*

1. **Ingredients:**
   - 1/4 cup dried goldenseal root
   - 1 cup carrier oil (e.g., olive oil, jojoba oil)
2. **Preparation:**
   - Place the dried goldenseal root in a clean glass jar.
   - Cover the roots completely with your chosen carrier oil.
   - Seal the jar tightly and place it in a warm, sunny spot for 4-6 weeks to infuse. Shake the jar gently every few days to ensure the roots are fully submerged.
3. **Straining and Storing:**
   - After infusion, strain the goldenseal-infused oil through a

fine mesh strainer or cheesecloth
into a clean container.

- Store the infused oil in a cool,
  dark place. Use it as a base for
  ointments or apply directly to the
  skin as needed for its
  antibacterial and healing benefits.

This goldenseal-infused oil recipe harnesses
the herb's potent antibacterial properties,
making it a valuable addition to your natural
first aid kit for promoting skin health and
supporting wound healing.

Marigold (Calendula officinalis)

Description: Marigold, scientifically known as Calendula officinalis, is a bright and cheerful flowering plant belonging to the Asteraceae family. Native to Mediterranean regions, it is cultivated globally for its ornamental beauty and medicinal properties. Marigold is characterized by its vibrant yellow or orange flowers and has a rich history of use in traditional medicine and skincare.

Scientific Benefits: Marigold contains beneficial compounds such as flavonoids (e.g., quercetin and luteolin), carotenoids (e.g., lutein and beta-carotene), and saponins. These constituents contribute to marigold's anti-inflammatory, antioxidant, and antimicrobial properties. Marigold is revered for its ability to soothe skin irritations, promote wound healing, and support overall skin health.

Antibacterial Properties: Marigold exhibits mild to moderate antibacterial activity against various bacteria, including both Gram-positive (e.g., Staphylococcus aureus) and Gram-negative (e.g., Escherichia coli) strains. The presence of flavonoids and other bioactive compounds in marigold helps inhibit bacterial growth and protect against infections.

Types of Infections Targeted: Marigold is effective in treating and soothing various topical infections and skin conditions:

- **Minor Wounds and Cuts:** Applied topically, marigold accelerates wound healing by reducing inflammation, stimulating tissue regeneration, and preventing infection.
- **Skin Irritations:** It provides relief for irritated skin, making it beneficial for conditions such as eczema, dermatitis, and minor burns.
- **Acne:** Marigold's antibacterial properties can help alleviate acne symptoms by combating surface bacteria and promoting skin clarity.

Dosage Recommendations: For topical use, marigold can be prepared in different forms, including infused oils, salves, and compresses. Use as directed on product labels or consult with a healthcare provider for specific dosage recommendations.

Preparation Recipe: *Marigold Salve:*

1. **Ingredients:**

- 1/4 cup dried marigold flowers (or fresh petals)
  - 1/2 cup coconut oil
  - 1 tablespoon beeswax pellets

2. **Preparation:**
   - In a double boiler or a heat-safe bowl placed over a pot of simmering water, combine the coconut oil and dried marigold flowers.
   - Heat gently for 1-2 hours to infuse the oil with the marigold's beneficial compounds. Stir occasionally and maintain low heat to avoid overheating.
   - Strain the infused oil using a fine mesh strainer or cheesecloth into a clean bowl.

3. **Adding Beeswax:**
   - Return the strained infused oil to the double boiler or heat-safe bowl.
   - Add beeswax pellets to the infused oil and stir continuously until the beeswax is completely melted and well combined with the oil.

4. **Cooling and Storing:**

- o   Pour the mixture into clean, dry containers or jars.
- o   Let the salve cool and solidify at room temperature before sealing the containers.
- o   Store the marigold salve in a cool, dark place. Apply topically as needed to soothe skin irritations, promote wound healing, and benefit from its antibacterial properties.

This marigold salve recipe offers a practical and effective way to harness the herb's antibacterial and healing properties, making it an excellent addition to your natural skincare routine for promoting healthy and radiant skin.

Comfrey (Symphytum officinale)

Description: Comfrey, scientifically known as Symphytum officinale, is a perennial herb native to Europe and parts of Asia. It belongs to the Boraginaceae family and is characterized by its robust, hairy stems and broad, lance-shaped leaves. Comfrey has a long history of use in traditional medicine for its healing properties, earning it the nickname "knitbone" due to its ability to promote bone and tissue healing.

Scientific Benefits: Comfrey contains various bioactive compounds, including allantoin, rosmarinic acid, and tannins. These constituents contribute to comfrey's anti-inflammatory, antioxidant, and wound-healing properties. Allantoin, in particular, stimulates cell proliferation and tissue regeneration, making comfrey effective in promoting skin health and accelerating wound healing.

Antibacterial Properties: Comfrey exhibits mild antibacterial activity against certain bacteria, primarily due to its allantoin content and other bioactive compounds. While not as potent as some other herbs, comfrey's antibacterial effects contribute to its overall wound-healing properties by protecting against infection.

Types of Infections Targeted: Comfrey is particularly beneficial for treating and soothing various skin conditions and injuries:

- **Wound Healing:** Applied topically, comfrey promotes the healing of cuts, bruises, and minor wounds by reducing inflammation, stimulating tissue repair, and protecting against infection.
- **Burns and Scalds:** Its soothing and emollient properties make comfrey useful in treating minor burns and scalds, providing relief and supporting skin regeneration.
- **Skin Irritations:** Comfrey ointments or poultices can help alleviate symptoms of eczema, dermatitis, and insect bites due to its calming and anti-inflammatory effects.

Dosage Recommendations: For topical use, comfrey is commonly applied in the form of creams, ointments, or poultices. Follow product-specific instructions or consult with a healthcare provider for appropriate dosage and application recommendations.

Preparation Recipe: *Comfrey Poultice:*

1. **Ingredients:**
   - Fresh comfrey leaves (or dried comfrey leaf powder)
   - Warm water
   - Optional: Cloth or gauze for wrapping
2. **Preparation:**
   - If using fresh comfrey leaves, crush or chop them finely to release their juices. If using dried comfrey leaf powder, mix it with enough warm water to form a thick paste.
   - Apply the comfrey paste directly to the affected area of the skin, ensuring a thick, even layer.
   - Cover the poultice with a clean cloth or gauze to keep it in place.
3. **Application:**
   - Leave the comfrey poultice on the skin for 30 minutes to 1 hour, or as directed by your healthcare provider.
   - Remove the poultice and gently rinse the area with warm water.
   - Repeat the application as needed to support wound healing and alleviate skin irritations.

Hyssop (Hyssopus officinalis)

Description: Hyssop, scientifically known as Hyssopus officinalis, is a herbaceous plant belonging to the Lamiaceae family, native to Southern Europe, the Middle East, and parts of Asia. It is characterized by its upright stems, narrow leaves, and clusters of small, fragrant blue or purple flowers. Hyssop has a long history of use in traditional medicine and culinary practices, prized for its aromatic properties and medicinal benefits.

Scientific Benefits: Hyssop contains several bioactive compounds, including volatile oils (e.g., pinocamphone, isopinocamphone), flavonoids, and tannins. These constituents contribute to hyssop's medicinal properties, including its anti-inflammatory, antioxidant, and antimicrobial effects. Hyssop is valued for its ability to support respiratory health, aid digestion, and promote skin wellness.

Antibacterial Properties: Hyssop exhibits moderate antibacterial activity against various bacteria, including both Gram-positive (e.g., Staphylococcus aureus) and Gram-negative (e.g., Escherichia coli) strains. The volatile oils in hyssop, particularly pinocamphone and isopinocamphone, are responsible for its antimicrobial effects, which help inhibit bacterial growth and protect against infections.

Types of Infections Targeted: Hyssop is beneficial for treating and soothing various topical infections and skin conditions:

- **Respiratory Infections:** Inhalation of hyssop vapors or use in steam inhalations can help alleviate symptoms of respiratory infections such as coughs, colds, and bronchitis.
- **Skin Irritations:** Applied topically, hyssop-infused oils or ointments can help reduce inflammation and soothe skin irritations, including minor cuts, scrapes, and insect bites.
- **Digestive Issues:** Hyssop teas or extracts are used traditionally to aid digestion, alleviate gastrointestinal discomfort, and support overall digestive health.

Dosage Recommendations: For topical applications, hyssop can be prepared in various forms, including infused oils, ointments, and compresses. Follow product-specific instructions or consult with a healthcare provider for appropriate dosage and application recommendations.

Preparation Recipe: *Hyssop Infused Oil:*

1. **Ingredients:**
   - 1/4 cup dried hyssop leaves and flowers
   - 1 cup carrier oil (e.g., olive oil, almond oil)
2. **Preparation:**
   - Place the dried hyssop leaves and flowers in a clean glass jar.
   - Cover the herbs completely with your chosen carrier oil.
   - Seal the jar tightly and place it in a warm, sunny spot for 4-6 weeks to infuse. Shake the jar gently every few days to ensure the herbs are fully submerged.
3. **Straining and Storing:**
   - After infusion, strain the hyssop-infused oil through a fine mesh strainer or cheesecloth into a clean container.
   - Store the infused oil in a cool, dark place. Use it as a base for ointments or apply directly to the skin as needed for its antibacterial and soothing properties.

Lemon Balm (Melissa officinalis)

Description: Lemon Balm, scientifically known as Melissa officinalis, is a perennial herb belonging to the Lamiaceae family. Native to the Mediterranean region, lemon balm is characterized by its lemon-scented leaves and small white or pale pink flowers. It has a long history of use in traditional medicine, culinary arts, and aromatherapy due to its pleasant fragrance and therapeutic properties.

Scientific Benefits: Lemon Balm contains several bioactive compounds, including volatile oils (e.g., citronellal, citral), polyphenols (e.g., rosmarinic acid), and flavonoids. These constituents contribute to lemon balm's medicinal properties, which include anti-inflammatory, antioxidant, antimicrobial, and calming effects. Lemon balm is valued for its ability to promote relaxation, support digestive health, and soothe skin irritations.

Antibacterial Properties: Lemon Balm exhibits mild to moderate antibacterial activity against various bacteria, including both Gram-positive (e.g., Staphylococcus aureus) and Gram-negative (e.g., Escherichia coli) strains. The volatile oils and polyphenols in lemon balm contribute to its antimicrobial effects, helping to inhibit bacterial growth and protect against infections.

Types of Infections Targeted: Lemon Balm is beneficial for treating and soothing various topical infections and skin conditions:

- **Cold Sores (Herpes Simplex Virus):** Topical application of lemon balm cream or ointment may help reduce the severity and duration of cold sores caused by the herpes simplex virus.
- **Skin Irritations:** Lemon balm-infused oils or creams can help alleviate symptoms of minor skin irritations, including itching, redness, and inflammation.
- **Wound Healing:** Its antimicrobial and anti-inflammatory properties support wound healing processes by protecting against infection and promoting skin regeneration.

Dosage Recommendations: For topical use, lemon balm can be applied in the form of creams, ointments, or infused oils. Follow product-specific instructions or consult with a healthcare provider for appropriate dosage and application recommendations.

Preparation Recipe: *Lemon Balm Infused Oil:*

1. **Ingredients:**
    - 1/2 cup dried lemon balm leaves
    - 1 cup carrier oil (e.g., olive oil, jojoba oil)
2. **Preparation:**

- o   Place the dried lemon balm leaves in a clean glass jar.
- o   Cover the leaves completely with your chosen carrier oil.
- o   Seal the jar tightly and place it in a warm, sunny spot for 4-6 weeks to infuse. Shake the jar gently every few days to ensure the leaves are fully submerged.

3. **Straining and Storing:**
- o   After infusion, strain the lemon balm-infused oil through a fine mesh strainer or cheesecloth into a clean container.
- o   Store the infused oil in a cool, dark place. Use it as a base for creams, lotions, or apply directly to the skin as needed for its antibacterial and soothing properties.

This lemon balm-infused oil recipe provides a natural and gentle solution for harnessing the herb's antibacterial and skin-soothing benefits in topical applications, supporting overall skin health and promoting natural healing processes.

Mullein (Verbascum thapsus)

Description: Mullein, scientifically known as Verbascum thapsus, is a biennial herbaceous plant native to Europe, Asia, and North Africa, now widely naturalized in temperate regions worldwide. It belongs to the Scrophulariaceae family and is characterized by its tall, erect stem covered with dense, soft hairs and large, velvety leaves. Mullein has a history of traditional medicinal use, especially for respiratory and skin ailments.

Scientific Benefits: Mullein contains various bioactive compounds such as saponins, mucilage, flavonoids, and iridoids. These constituents contribute to its medicinal properties, including anti-inflammatory, antioxidant, expectorant, and mild antimicrobial effects. Mullein is renowned for its ability to support respiratory health, soothe mucous membranes, and aid skin wellness.

Antibacterial Properties: While primarily known for its soothing and respiratory benefits, mullein also exhibits mild antibacterial activity. This is attributed to its saponins and other bioactive compounds, which help inhibit bacterial growth and promote skin healing.

Types of Infections Targeted: Mullein is beneficial for treating and soothing various infections and conditions:

- **Respiratory Infections:** Helps relieve symptoms of coughs, bronchitis, and congestion by reducing inflammation and supporting respiratory function.
- **Ear Infections:** Topically applied mullein oil can alleviate pain and inflammation associated with ear infections and aid in reducing bacterial presence in the ear canal.
- **Skin Irritations:** Mullein-infused oils or ointments soothe minor cuts, burns, and insect bites due to their anti-inflammatory and emollient properties.

Dosage Recommendations: For topical applications, mullein can be used in various forms such as oils, ointments, and compresses. Follow product-specific instructions or consult with a healthcare provider for appropriate dosage and application recommendations.

Compress Recipe: *Mullein Leaf Compress:*

1. **Ingredients:**
    - 1 cup dried mullein leaves (or fresh leaves)
    - 2 cups boiling water
    - Clean cloth or gauze
2. **Preparation:**
    - Place the dried mullein leaves (or fresh leaves) in a heatproof bowl.
    - Pour the boiling water over the leaves, enough to fully submerge them.

- Let the mixture steep for 10-15 minutes to allow the beneficial compounds to infuse into the water.

3. **Application:**
   - Dip a clean cloth or gauze into the mullein-infused water, allowing it to soak up the liquid.
   - Wring out excess liquid from the cloth (while still keeping it moist).
   - Apply the warm, moist compress directly to the affected area of the skin (e.g., on a wound, rash, or inflamed area).

4. **Duration:**
   - Leave the compress in place for 15-20 minutes, or as directed by your healthcare provider.
   - Reapply the compress as needed to help soothe and promote healing.

This mullein leaf compress recipe offers a natural and gentle way to harness the herb's antibacterial and healing benefits for topical applications, supporting overall skin health and aiding in the recovery from minor skin irritations and injuries.

Plantain (Plantago major)

Description: Plantain, scientifically known as Plantago major, is a perennial herbaceous plant native to Europe and now naturalized throughout temperate regions worldwide. Belonging to the Plantaginaceae family, it is characterized by its low-growing rosette of broad, oval-shaped leaves and slender, greenish flower spikes. Despite its name, plantain is not related to the banana-like fruit but is highly valued for its medicinal properties.

Scientific Benefits: Plantain contains several bioactive compounds, including aucubin, allantoin, flavonoids, and tannins. These constituents contribute to its medicinal properties, which include anti-inflammatory, antimicrobial, and wound-healing effects. Plantain is known for its ability to soothe irritated skin, promote tissue repair, and support overall skin health.

Antibacterial Properties: Plantain exhibits mild to moderate antibacterial activity against various bacteria, including both Gram-positive (e.g., Staphylococcus aureus) and Gram-negative (e.g., Escherichia coli) strains. The presence of aucubin and other bioactive compounds contributes to its antimicrobial effects, helping to inhibit bacterial growth and protect against infections.

Types of Infections Targeted: Plantain is beneficial for treating and soothing various topical infections and skin conditions:

- **Wound Healing:** Applied topically, plantain helps promote wound healing by reducing inflammation, accelerating tissue regeneration, and protecting against infection.
- **Skin Irritations:** It provides relief for minor skin irritations such as insect bites, rashes, and minor burns, due to its soothing and anti-inflammatory properties.
- **Acne:** Plantain's antimicrobial effects can help reduce acne symptoms by combating surface bacteria and supporting clearer skin.

Dosage Recommendations: For topical use, plantain can be prepared in various forms, including poultices, creams, and infused oils. Follow product-specific instructions or consult with a healthcare provider for appropriate dosage and application recommendations.

Preparation Recipe: *Plantain Poultice:*

1. **Ingredients:**
    - Fresh plantain leaves (washed and chopped)
    - Warm water (optional)
    - Clean cloth or gauze
2. **Preparation:**

- Crush or chop fresh plantain leaves to release their juices and active compounds.
   - If desired, heat the leaves briefly in warm water to soften them and enhance their medicinal properties.
   - Place the crushed leaves directly onto the affected area of the skin.
3. **Application:**
   - Cover the plantain leaves with a clean cloth or gauze to keep them in place.
   - Leave the poultice on the skin for 20-30 minutes, or as directed by your healthcare provider.
   - Remove the poultice and gently rinse the area with warm water.
4. **Repeat as Needed:**
   - Repeat the plantain poultice application as often as necessary to soothe skin irritations, promote healing, and support overall skin health.

This plantain poultice recipe offers a natural and effective way to harness the herb's antibacterial and healing properties for topical applications, providing relief and promoting skin wellness.

St. John's Wort (Hypericum perforatum)

Description: St. John's Wort, scientifically known as Hypericum perforatum, is a flowering plant native to Europe, Asia, and parts of Africa, but it is now naturalized in many parts of the world. It belongs to the Hypericaceae family and is characterized by its bright yellow flowers and perforated leaves, from which it derives its scientific name. St. John's Wort has a long history of use in herbal medicine for its antidepressant, anti-inflammatory, and wound-healing properties.

Scientific Benefits: St. John's Wort contains several bioactive compounds, including hypericin, hyperforin, flavonoids (such as quercetin and rutin), and tannins. These constituents contribute to its medicinal properties, which include antidepressant, anti-inflammatory, antimicrobial, and wound-healing effects. St. John's Wort is known for its ability to improve mood, reduce inflammation, and promote skin health.

Antibacterial Properties: St. John's Wort exhibits mild antibacterial activity against certain bacteria, primarily attributed to its hyperforin content and other bioactive compounds. While not as potent as some other herbs, its antimicrobial effects contribute to its overall therapeutic benefits, especially in supporting skin health and wound healing.

Types of Infections Targeted: St. John's Wort is beneficial for treating and soothing various skin infections and conditions:

- **Wound Healing:** Applied topically, St. John's Wort helps accelerate wound healing by reducing inflammation, promoting tissue regeneration, and protecting against infection.
- **Minor Burns and Sunburns:** Its soothing and anti-inflammatory properties provide relief for minor burns and sunburns, supporting skin recovery and reducing discomfort.
- **Herpes Simplex Virus:** Topical application of St. John's Wort oil or ointment may help reduce the severity and duration of cold sores caused by the herpes simplex virus.

Dosage Recommendations: For topical use, St. John's Wort can be prepared in various forms, including infused oils, creams, and ointments. Follow product-specific instructions or consult with a healthcare provider for appropriate dosage and application recommendations.

Preparation Recipe: *St. John's Wort Infused Oil:*

1. **Ingredients:**
    - 1/2 cup dried St. John's Wort flowers and leaves

- 1 cup carrier oil (e.g., olive oil, coconut oil)

2. **Preparation:**
   - Place the dried St. John's Wort flowers and leaves in a clean glass jar.
   - Cover the herbs completely with your chosen carrier oil.
   - Seal the jar tightly and place it in a warm, sunny spot for 4-6 weeks to infuse. Shake the jar gently every few days to ensure the herbs are fully submerged.

3. **Straining and Storing:**
   - After infusion, strain the St. John's Wort-infused oil through a fine mesh strainer or cheesecloth into a clean container.
   - Store the infused oil in a cool, dark place. Use it as a base for creams, ointments, or apply directly to the skin as needed for its antibacterial and soothing properties.

This St. John's Wort-infused oil recipe provides a natural and gentle way to harness the herb's antibacterial and healing benefits for topical applications, supporting overall skin health and promoting natural healing processes.

Yarrow (Achillea millefolium)

Description: Yarrow, scientifically known as Achillea millefolium, is a flowering perennial herb belonging to the Asteraceae family. Native to Europe and Asia, yarrow is now naturalized and widely cultivated in temperate regions around the world. It is characterized by its feathery, fern-like leaves and flat-topped clusters of small white, pink, or yellow flowers. Yarrow has a rich history of use in traditional medicine and herbal remedies due to its diverse medicinal properties.

Scientific Benefits: Yarrow contains bioactive compounds such as flavonoids (e.g., apigenin, luteolin), sesquiterpene lactones, tannins, and volatile oils. These constituents contribute to yarrow's medicinal properties, including anti-inflammatory, antimicrobial, astringent, and wound-healing effects. Yarrow is valued for its ability to promote circulation, reduce inflammation, and support overall skin health.

Antibacterial Properties: Yarrow exhibits significant antibacterial activity against various bacteria, both Gram-positive (e.g., Staphylococcus aureus) and Gram-negative (e.g., Escherichia coli) strains. The presence of flavonoids and volatile oils contributes to its antimicrobial effects, helping to inhibit bacterial growth and protect against infections.

Types of Infections Targeted: Yarrow is beneficial for treating and soothing various skin infections and conditions:

- **Wound Healing:** Applied topically, yarrow promotes wound healing by stimulating tissue repair, reducing inflammation, and preventing infection.
- **Minor Cuts and Scrapes:** Its antiseptic and astringent properties help cleanse wounds, reduce bleeding, and accelerate healing.
- **Skin Irritations:** Yarrow-infused oils or ointments can soothe skin irritations, including rashes, eczema, and insect bites, due to its anti-inflammatory and calming effects.

Dosage Recommendations: For topical use, yarrow can be prepared in various forms, including poultices, infused oils, and ointments. Follow product-specific instructions or consult with a healthcare provider for appropriate dosage and application recommendations.

Preparation Recipe: *Yarrow Infused Oil:*

1. **Ingredients:**
   - 1/2 cup dried yarrow flowers and leaves
   - 1 cup carrier oil (e.g., olive oil, almond oil)
2. **Preparation:**

- Place the dried yarrow flowers and leaves in a clean glass jar.
- Cover the herbs completely with your chosen carrier oil.
- Seal the jar tightly and place it in a warm, sunny spot for 4-6 weeks to infuse. Shake the jar gently every few days to ensure the herbs are fully submerged.

3. **Straining and Storing:**
- After infusion, strain the yarrow-infused oil through a fine mesh strainer or cheesecloth into a clean container.
- Store the infused oil in a cool, dark place. Use it as a base for ointments, creams, or apply directly to the skin as needed for its antibacterial and soothing properties.

This yarrow-infused oil recipe provides a natural and effective way to harness the herb's antibacterial and healing benefits for topical applications, supporting overall skin health and aiding in the relief of various skin conditions and irritations.